THE BUSY

PRINCIPLES FOR BUILDING A GREAT PHYSIQUE WITHOUT MISSING OUT ON LIFE

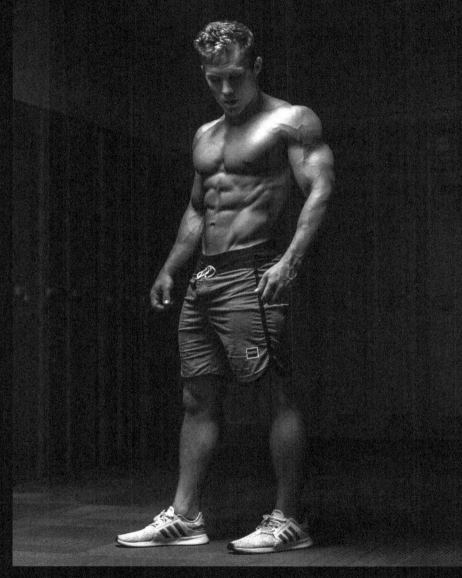

JOHN DELUCA, RN, BSN, CCRN

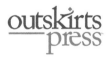

"Do not go gentle into that good night,

Old age should burn and rave at close of day;

Rage, rage against the dying of the light."

- Dylan Thomas

Table of Contents

Trigger Warning

Be advised; this book is not for the faint of heart. If you're looking for someone to pat your belly and say you look awesome after sucking down your fifth Haagen-Dazs pint of the weekend, then I'm afraid we need to part ways now. While I would never intentionally hurl inflammatory comments at non-soliciting parties, I do wholeheartedly believe in putting honesty above kindness, and that lying as a means for protecting someone's feelings is still lying.

Adam Carolla made a profound speech to the US Congress in July 2018 where he likened the current "safe space" culture on college campuses to astronauts living inside the International Space Station for extended periods of time. Carolla explained that by not exposing these young adults to the harsh realities of the world, universities were raising them in a "zero-gravity bubble," wherein they were losing emotional fortitude in the same way that astronauts lose bone mass.

You are not entering a zero-gravity bubble by picking up this book.

I loathe body-shaming of any kind, and hold no disdain toward anyone who does not or cannot make fitness a priority. If you are but a casual passerby looking for some light reading, then rest assured that absolutely none of the disparaging comments to follow are directed at you. Keep living your life and being happy on your own terms.

However, if you have been present (very deliberate wording) in the gym for five hours a week over the last half decade and place the blame of your stagnation at the feet of poor genetics, bad weather, or the freaking Vietnam War, then you sir, are free game. For several of you circus clowns, the only change to your body during that span has been the loosely correlated scatterplot of crab grass speckled onto your cheeks which you've been tragically referring to as a beard. My taking it easy on you is only going to perpetuate this cycle. It's also not nearly as fun.

Socrates once proclaimed: "No man has the right to be an amateur in the matter of physical training. It is a shame for a man to grow old without seeing the beauty and strength of which his body is capable." *The Busy Body* will unlock all of the information you need to transform your physique and shove it down that old geezer's throat. Let us begin.

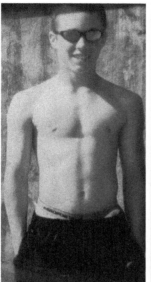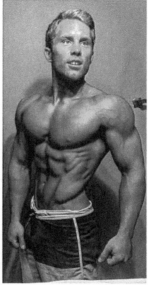

5 year process

On the left is a picture of me at fifteen years old. If you can manage to see through the sparkling white abyss that even the late Ray Charles would have a tough time staring at, you'll notice that my chest has the density of your standard 8.5x11 loose leaf sheet of paper. Or perhaps you'll notice that my shoulders are about as thick as a hot bowl of tap water. I could have walked buck naked and covered in steak sauce through a gaggle of starving cannibals without so much as raising an eyebrow. I spent the next five years sculpting and building the physique you see on the right.

Contrary to what you may believe, it wasn't all that difficult. I spent about six hours a week at the gym. I never obsessed over counting calories or a specific number of reps. I worked full time in the summers, averaged twenty hours per semester, and had plenty of time for concerts and ski trips. If forced to give my best estimate on the number of beers I consumed between these two still shots, the figure would be somewhere north of three thousand. I also never used any form of steroid, testosterone booster, or anything that you couldn't pick up

Still able to drink

from the local Vitamin Shoppe. So why then do I look so different from everyone else doing the same thing? Because of the specific strategies I am about to share with you that target and harass muscle bellies faster and more methodically than anything you've ever tried. I've probably been lifting a bit more than you, but what's far more consequential is that I've been lifting more EFFECTIVELY than you.

The Busy Body is not for someone looking to be the next Simeon Panda or Callum Von Moger. These are full-time athletes with some of the best physiques on the planet. If attaining their frame is your goal, go buy their program, stock up on illegal hormone concoctions, and say goodbye to your social life for the next two decades. Otherwise—and I cannot stress this enough—you have a ZERO percent chance of resembling these men. Then again, if you want to clock fifty hours a week at the office, grab some wings and a couple of beers on Friday night, and still turn heads at the pool the next day, then *The Busy Body* is precisely what you're looking for. ← Big seller (Relatable)

Maybe you've been lifting for years and can't seem to break through a plateau. Perhaps you're a former distance runner and now looking to pack on some size. Better yet, maybe you spent the last four years of college slurping down enough mop-bucket liquor and extended-release Adderall to send a full-grown African rhino to an early grave. Despite the fact that you were Honorable Mention All-Conference in high school football, you now run a ten-minute mile, your waist line is growing in dog years, and you cause a barren womb every time you cross the vicinity of an attractive woman. Face it, you're disgusting.

You may even be a forty-five-year-old dad trying to get back in the groove. Twenty years ago, you were the man: lean, confident, and full of life. Now you're shaped like a giant pear with legs. Your ancestors stalked prey for days at a time, staving off attacks from Comanche Indians and coyotes all the while. The only thing you've been stalking is the cheesecake line at the Golden Corral.

It's time to wake up. It's time to take back control of your body and return those testosterone levels to where they belong. You don't need someone to sugar coat it (or else you'd eat it LOL). Whether you know it or not, you need someone to crack your jaw with a closed-fist sucker punch filled with the God's honest truth. If you're looking for a twelve-week summer shred program, this ain't it. But if you want a set of principles you can stick with for decades, and build an aesthetic, functional physique without sacrificing your life to the iron gods, then read on.

Delivering
a "set of principle"
to the audience

Understanding Time

Before I divulge all of my secrets for efficiently building lean muscle, we have to get on the same page regarding the most indispensable aspect of anyone's fitness journey: time. The most common excuse I hear for why someone has let themselves mutate into a sweaty, mangy wilde-beest who gets winded squeezing into their favorite pair of cargo jorts is that they simply cannot carve out enough time in their busy sched-ules to make any progress in the gym. I used to think these people were just lazy. Rotting heaps of garbage. Literal pond scum. A complete waste of space and oxygen. I looked upon them with scorn, like a leper in the streets of ancient Babylon.

Saner thoughts prevailed, however, as I soon realized that the reason people can't find that one extra hour of time for the gym is because of a compilation of small blocks of wasted time throughout the day. They're spending an extra seven minutes in the shower after they've washed off, an additional nineteen minutes scrolling through Twitter memes after work, twenty-three minutes making sure their dinner is cooked to perfection, forty-two minutes for one more episode of *Breaking Bad*. I became OBSESSED with saving these small increments of time spent on menial tasks that provided me with menial levels of enjoyment.

Decide what is most important to you. Write down a handful of your favorite activities that bring you at least an eight out of ten on the happiness scale. Mine are skiing, golf, metal concerts, and sand volleyball. I would NEVER miss one of these for the gym, and would never expect you to either. Maybe you love hiking, collecting antiquated jazz vinyls, or selling organic cat food at Elizabeth Warren rallies. Whatever the case may be, you have to prioritize these high-enjoyment activities while considerably reducing the time you spend on things that bring you to a five or six on the happiness scale, such as swiping through bug-eyed, horoscope fanatics on Tinder. You may be surprised at how much extra time you can find in your schedule once you trim the fat, so to speak. I'm not saying to cut out all social media and movie time from your lives, but how interesting is your Facebook feed anyways? Oh my God, Tammy's having another baby and Aaron went to Charleston for the weekend? Call the National Guard! We have to throw a parade!

You can absolutely maintain a social life, a job, and a well-built physique. What I cannot guarantee is that you can maintain a social life, a job, a well-built physique, and enough time to binge watch Game of Thrones twice a week. Decide what your priorities are, and adjust accordingly.

Squeeze-Surrender-Stretch

Bodybuilding is far more cerebral than many have been conditioned to believe; it's not just a bunch of chimps slinging weights around for no reason. Proper bodybuilding requires intense levels of concentration and a coordinated plan of assault. You've probably heard about the mind-muscle connection, the idea that a deep focus on the internal workings of your musculoskeletal system can produce exponentially better results in building your physique. It sounds like some kind of mushroom-tripping pseudoscience, but I promise you the feeling is tangible and the effects are unquestionable. To properly develop this connection, you must funnel every ounce of your focus into *contracting* an individual muscle rather than simply *moving* a weight. The weight is but an extension of your arm. All it can do is add resistance. The muscle fibers themselves are what *move* the weight. If you're doing lat pull-downs, for example, you shouldn't be thinking about pulling the bar to your chest; you should be trying to contract your back muscles so hard, and at such a cellular level, that the bar has no *choice* but to come down to your chest.

This contraction is referred to as the concentric phase of the movement, whereas the return from full flex to starting position is the eccentric phase. The individual muscle fibers you wish to target should commandeer your entire thought process throughout these concentric and eccentric portions.

It sounds obvious, but trust when I say that I watch dudes on the pull-down machine every day, flailing around like one of those inflatable car lot balloons. In a surprisingly impressive feat of flexibility, their backs are actually parallel to the ground at the peak of their concentric motion. It's incredible. And by incredible, I mean incredibly counterproductive. Not only do they look spastic, uncoordinated, and mildly autistic, they also look exactly how they looked three years ago. To say that progress is a foreign concept to these men is an understatement akin to claiming that Stalin was not a fan boy for capitalism.

The mind-muscle connection is also what will improve your ability to isolate muscle groups when performing compound movements. Do you ever feel like close-grip bench press uses more of your chest than your triceps, or that side-lateral raises tend to exhaust your traps more so than your actual deltoids? This is because you have yet to perfect this vital neurological connection. Start working on it now, and as you incorporate the other Busy Body principles, isolating muscles will reveal itself as an esteemed craft, and will quickly take your physique to the next level.

If you take one thing away from the book, let it be this: there is something truly transcendent about the mind-muscle connection. It will take you months or even years to fully grasp, but the sense of control you feel when you are entirely in charge of each muscle in your body is indescribable.

Developing a heightened mind-muscle connection can be drastically accelerated by adopting my framework of squeeze-surrender-stretch. Squeeze refers to the concentric phase, which you now understand as the flexing portion of a movement that shortens the muscle. The next time you do a set of preacher curls, close your eyes and envision

Excellent Visuals

Vivid

Vivid —
LOL

yourself diving directly into your bicep muscle fibers. Don't *move* the weight. *Squeeze* the fibers. Squeeze them all. Squeeze them as hard as you possibly can. Squeeze them like a reticulated python choking out a gazelle as it tries to gouge your eyes out. Squeeze them like you've got half a dab of toothpaste left in the tube, and in spite of the fact that your breath smells like you've been gargling a week's worth of Woody Harrelson's jock sweat, there's a chick in the other room looking to make out. You need that toothpaste, bro. So squeeze it. And when you're at the peak of the movement, squeeze even harder.

After holding this squeeze for a moment (VERY IMPORTANT), move on to the surrender, and begin the eccentric phase of the movement.

You must surrender to the weight. Relinquish your squeeze as slowly as you can, ferociously fighting gravity while still allowing it to overtake you, as you retreat to the starting position. When performed correctly, the surrender is the most difficult part of any exercise, and therefore the most critical. Your body so badly wants to run from the pain, begging you to stop fighting and fully relax all tension. The reason you have the biceps of a professional XBOX player, among a laundry list of other factors, is largely due to the fact that you have been giving in to this urge. Stay in the fight until the very moment you reach the starting position.

Here is where you focus on the stretch. Let the weight completely dominate you as it pulls your muscle fibers, ligaments, and tendons apart. This will create an excruciating burn that you will soon come to crave. For bicep curls, this is with arms fully extended. Block everything out except for the pain. Let the arms inch so close to flaccidity that the weight nearly falls from your fingers.

Muscle fibers are surrounded by a rigid layer of connective tissue, called fascia, which acts as a mechanical barrier to muscle expansion (Lee, 2007). Because this fibrous network of fascia is so tough, following

up each contraction with a skin splitting stretch is absolutely imperative if the underlying muscles are to have any chance at increasing in
size. Hany Rambod has trained more Mr. and Mrs. Olympia (the Super
Bowl equivalent of professional bodybuilding) champions than any other trainer in the world. FST-7 (Fascia stretch training) is his patented
system, and it has irrefutably produced better results than any fitness
program to date by means of an all-out, no-holds-barred Blitzkrieg of
this pesky layer of tissue.

Do be careful to differentiate between the rest position and the
stretch position, as these may be identical or opposite, depending on
the exercise. As mentioned above, the stretch position for preacher
curls is with the arms fully extended. Contrarily, the stretch position
for barbell bench press is with the elbows bent and the bar lying across
the chest. Wherever the proper stretch position may be, it should be
held for one to five seconds before beginning again with the squeeze.

You just performed a *single* quality repetition. If this felt distinctly more
intense than past efforts, then you are starting to understand why you
have been making tectonic-plate levels of progress. Consider this your
metamorphosis. Every solitary rep you perform from this point forward should feel as deliberate and as measured as this one.

There is a particular cadence to the squeeze-surrender-stretch method, and capturing it is essential, but may take some time. An easy way to
make this cadence become habit is to over-accentuate your breathing
pattern. Before beginning a set, take a massive nasal breath from your
diaphragm and hold. Exhale through the mouth just as you begin the
squeeze, blowing forcefully and steadily through pursed lips. Imagine
you are trying to blow out a candle sitting four feet in front of your
face. Your lungs should completely empty just as you finish the squeeze
and prepare to surrender. Now inhale through the nose once again,
starting and stopping the breath concurrently with the duration of the
surrender. Inhale as if a warm, errant protein fart inadvertently slipped

out just before picking up a hot date. You have to make absolutely certain that none of the ghastly remnants of your atrocious dietary habits are lingering before allowing this poor girl into your car, so you better sniff hard and deep. Finally, maintain the stretch position with a full set of lungs for as long as you can manage, and then repeat the entire process.

Forceful, oral exhale. Squeeze.

Deep, nasal inhale. Surrender.

Hold. Stretch. Repeat.

Executing this deep, rhythmic breathing style over the course of just a single set can very easily bring you to a euphoric, meditative state. As you enter this trance-like zone, allow the abundance of apprehensions circling your brain to silently drift away, leaving nothing but perception of this most immediate reality. Feel the air expanding your rib cage as sweat droplets amass on your forehead. Take note of the searing, but strangely satisfying burn emanating from your exhausting muscle tissue. Ignore the impulse to succumb as you bestow YOUR will upon the weight. Take yourself to the edge of your very existence. I realize it's a bit contradictory to receive meditation advice from a man who just referenced an ill-timed, aerial bowel release, but you got yourself into this mess buying my book, so I'm not sure what to tell you.

Hypertrophy vs. Strength

Force yourself to struggle (handwritten annotation)

To further facilitate your squeeze-surrender-stretch technique, try making the weight feel as *heavy* as possible in your brain. Force yourself to struggle with it, no matter if its 240 pounds or 12. Let's say you're finishing up chest day with some 30-pound flat bench dumbbell flies. You should be moving so purposefully and contracting so consciously that it feels like 100 pounds. Slow and controlled reps are the key. Feel each individual fiber contracting and releasing. Chase the burn and then live in it. Live in it until you reach the point of failure. You will be shocked at how sore this will make you, and how drastically it will shorten the length of your workouts due to sheer exhaustion. Simply put, if you're not thinking this way in the gym, you might as well stay home.

To fully grasp the concept of making the weight *heavy*, consider the dichotomy of bodybuilding, which is mainly hypertrophy-based training, and Olympic/powerlifting, which are instead strength-based training. These exercises are a completely different breed and are all about *explosion* rather than *contraction, strength* rather than *hypertrophy*. You *explode* into a clean and jerk. You *explode* into a heavy squat. You *explode* into a power snatch. If you want bigger deltoids, then you should be making lateral raises or military presses feel as *heavy* as possible.

Conversely, if your goal is to increase your one-rep max on deadlift, then you should be making the weight feel as *light* as possible, *exploding* off the ground with each rep.

I try to maintain a healthy ratio of bodybuilding to Olympic/powerlifting, both for fun and for functionality. Most workouts, after warming up, I spend anywhere from ten to twenty minutes on a heavy, compound movement (bench, squat, Arnold press, etc.) or Olympic lift (snatch, hang clean, etc.) to improve my strength before moving on to auxiliary/isolation movements that promote hypertrophy. Although several exercises can be performed in such a way that satisfies either category, there is nothing similar about the two styles, and you must completely shift your mindset when switching between them. Deadlift is one such example. You can explode with heavy-weight, low-rep sets to build strength, or you can use light/medium weight with higher rep counts to build defined muscle. If you squeeze, surrender, and stretch with 90 percent of your deadlift max, you will quickly become the first ever human being in recorded history to be airlifted out of a Planet Fitness, a remarkable achievement in its own right.

Just remember: liars do not get shredded. When you first start using the squeeze-surrender-stretch technique, you will feel weaker than ever before. This means you are executing correctly, but it also means that you have been cheating reps for your entire life. Use this as a catalyst for some genuine, soul-churning introspection. You won't get anywhere if you're not honest with yourself. Look back to my physique at fifteen. I was a card-carrying weasel. Had a stiff breeze hit me in an open field, I would have blown clear into the stratosphere. A few small changes implemented with consistency, and I was able to transform into that mega tool on the cover. You can make some serious progress over the next few years, but only if you are 100 percent brutally honest with yourself, and honesty in the weight room entails only grabbing weights that you can undeniably control.

Repeat after me: NO EGO LIFTING. Nobody cares if you can curl the 50s while rocking back and forth like some kind of rabid, silverback ape dodging tranquilizer darts. So stop trying to impress the sorority chick on the leg press machine; she has a boyfriend named Chad and his dad runs a law firm. Drop the weight and perform quality repetitions. Some days, I may never go above 25 pounds on bicep curls for an entire session. To fully engage the bicep and contract the muscle properly, the weight MUST be controllable. If 50 pounds is barely controllable for me, it almost certainly is not controllable for you, or else you would not be reading this book. You will get stronger, and when you do, the weights will increase, but first, we have to develop an ironclad mind-muscle connection. Do you want bigger, leaner biceps, or do you want to be able to curl the 50s? OK then, drop the weight.

Failure = Success

Anyone who has ever lifted (contracted muscles*) with me knows that I never count reps. Unless you are performing unilateral movements that must be reciprocated on the contralateral side, then rep counting will only get in your way. You should be so enthralled in *squeezing* your lats, or your pecs, or your rhomboids, or your calves that you can't possibly count. Counting reps forces you to either cheat your form in order to reach an arbitrarily named boundary, or creates a false ceiling which you WILL use to cut yourself short. Instead, you should be skirting along the line of failure, which I define as "losing the ability to perform quality reps with a full range of motion," multiple times throughout a single workout.

This is the key to making such tremendous progress in such a short period of time. Have a ballpark estimate of reps you want to reach *before* a set, and adjust the weight *between* sets accordingly. Once you start a set, however, you've committed to that weight. Destroy it. Take yourself to the edge. Find out EXACTLY where your breaking point is. Squeeze, surrender, and stretch until you simply cannot continue. However, as a point of caution, make sure to have a good spotter when approaching failure on any exercise that could put you in jeopardy of physical harm, such as bench press or squat. Nobody wants to run over to save your sweaty ass from the ensuing aneurysm in the middle of their set.

Dorian Yates won six consecutive Mr. Olympia titles during the height of his bodybuilding career. From 1992 to 1997, there was not a soul on planet Earth that was more capable at packing on muscle and eliminating fat than Dorian Yates. His wins are impressive no doubt, but his contribution to the competitive bodybuilding world far surpassed his trophy collection, as he is perhaps most known for the notoriously short duration of his workouts. His high-intensity training strategies, focused on minimal repetitions with maximal effort, caused a paradigm shift that rang throughout the entire fitness industry, as there was now demonstrable evidence that building a great physique did not require endless hours of grueling repetition. His basic premise was to perform three to four warm-up sets with each exercise before taking a SINGLE working set to absolute failure.

In a 2019 interview with Bodybuilding.com, Yates explained, "If you complete that one set to failure and push it to the absolute limit, that is going to be sufficient stimulus and intensity. So doing it again is not really going to give you anything additional and might possibly be more stress for your body to recover from, so it may be harder to recover, and without recovery you are not going to grow."

Yates was obviously using copious amounts of drugs to achieve his massive size, but that does not make his theories null and void for the common man. Going to failure is a crucial element to stimulating muscle growth in the midst of a busy life, and has been a staple of my routines for years. However, it was not until I began expanding my set past the point of failure by way of the drop set that I fully understood what it meant to reach exhaustion.

Drop sets have the unique ability to turn an otherwise mediocre workout into an unlicensed, bareknuckle death match, the likes of which Tyler Durden himself would willingly ascend down from Lou's Sky Tavern to partake. Let's say I'm doing DB lateral raises to finish off my shoulders. I might start with eight to twenty reps with the 35s, or as many as I can until I approach failure. As soon as I rerack the 35s, I'm picking up the 20s, and I'm right back at it for as many as I can handle. When I can't perform another quality rep, I rerack the 20s, and immediately grab the 8s for another burnout.

By this point, I'm in a raw, primal state. Foam is beginning to accumulate at the edges of my mouth. I've sprouted fangs. My face is purple. My visual spectrum has expanded to the point that I can now perceive ultraviolet and infrared light waves. My exoskeleton has been shed and my soul now floats above my body. My delts feel like they've been smothered in molten lava. I'm sweating like a middle school boy whose mom just discovered his vintage porn collection. This place is everything to me. If you wish to possess a hard, well-built physique in the midst of a busy schedule, then you must learn to love this place.

Notice that, by the end of my example, I was using the 8 pound weights. As of this writing, my old man is half way to a hundred and thirty years old. He was around when they invented dirt. He's got two fake knees, seven heart stents, half a prostate, and is about as flexible as a Hemlock two-by-four. Even still, he can eat the 8 pound dumbbells as an hors devoirs. So then why would I, a 24-year-old physical specimen in the prime of his life, associate myself with such an insultingly light weight? Because I am not a child. I have no interest in looking cool for the Division 2 frat star vape-lords snapping mirror pics by the Smith machine. I am here to improve my physique by any means necessary, and that is all.

7x Mr. Olympia champion, Arnold Schwarzenegger, has remained a vocal advocate for the drop set throughout his career, and attributes much of his success to this very concept. In the famed 1970s film Pumping Iron, Arnold shares his technique of "running the rack", in which he would start with a single bicep curl using the heaviest weight he could manage, and then drop up to ten different times to complete his first of several sets. He didn't give a rat's ass about how he looked near the end of his sets, struggling with weights that he could ordinarily toss through the ceiling; he was merely chasing the pump, and you would be wise to follow suit.

Superset for Super Gains

Going to failure like this obviously requires some recuperation time between sets. You can either pull out your phone to scroll through the plethora of brain-numbingly superficial trash collections that make up your Instagram feed, or you can take a *working* rest by way of an antagonist superset. This involves combining two different exercises of opposing body parts which you alternate between for several sets. For example, let's say I'm hitting back and triceps. I might hit a set of neutral grip narrow pulldowns for my lats and rhomboids. After approaching or reaching failure, I immediately move on to overhead rope extensions for my triceps. During this set, my back is completely uninvolved and can recover a bit while my triceps take on the workload. As soon as I approach or reach failure on rope extensions, I immediately move back to the pulldowns, where my now-exhausted triceps can take their much needed rest.

I will oscillate between these two motions anywhere from three to ten times, depending on how it feels, adjusting the weights up or down to suit my preference. Remember not to fixate on a specific rep range or number of sets. Focus on the burn. Squeeze, surrender, and stretch with every single rep. I've gotten myself into such a good zone before that I performed this exact superset for my entire workout. I was so sore that I couldn't wash between my shoulder blades for a week. It was glorious.

For antagonist supersets to work as intended, you MUST fully isolate the opposing muscle groups involved in the rotation. This is why developing your mind-muscle connection is such a central pillar in *The Busy Body*. While one group is working, the other is RESTING. The triceps extensions in this example are supposed to be as taxing for the lats as merely resting on the bench. You've just taken your lats to failure, and are moments away from repeating the process. If you don't develop a strong mind-muscle connection, then actually resting them while taking your triceps to failure will be impossible.

There are differing opinions on this topic. Some feel as though you should superset two cooperating body parts, such as back and biceps, or chest and triceps. So instead of the rope extensions in the previous example, one might alternate between the pulldowns, which already involve the biceps, and kettlebell curls, which use only the biceps. However, because your biceps get zero time to recuperate during this evolution, you will invariably sacrifice form and reach exhaustion substantially earlier, leaving your lats hungry for more. Your arms may get a 9/10 pump, but because the biceps are so fatigued, your back pump may only reach a 4/10. To each their own, but using *opposing* rather than *cooperating* muscle groups has worked best for me. ← To each their own

Nevertheless, the continual movement brought about by any superset will significantly increase your heart rate, abetting fat loss and improving your cardiovascular endurance in much more amusing and efficient means than merely jogging on a treadmill. Like most of you, I work full time, I love to travel, and I will always prioritize spending time with friends and family. I don't have time to spend an hour lifting weights and thirty minutes doing cardio every day. With *The Busy Body* principles, and particularly the antagonist superset, I am able to COMBINE my weight training with my fat burning, saving precious moments of time that I can spend on the things I love most.

When you're really ready to get nasty, you can combine your supersets with your drop sets, a "super drop" if you will. Perform a drop set as described above. Upon completion of your final drop, move on to an opposing muscle movement and perform another drop set, repeating the entire process several times over. I am certainly no expert in the field of Eastern Religion, but I can confidently assume that when Buddha spoke of nirvana, he was referring to the super drop.

Twist that Wrist

Eventually, your body will adapt to this repetitive trauma, and if you do not switch up your routines, then your progress will slow to a halt. You can stay ahead of your body's natural adaptation by implementing the often-trivialized, but ever-so-essential concept of grip variation. Everyone knows they should work on wide, narrow, and shoulder-width hand spacing on any exercise that will allow it. However, too often dismissed or ignored altogether is wrist rotation. For almost any free weight exercise, two to three wrist variations can be applied, each targeting specific areas of a muscle belly.

Neutral grip, also commonly referred to as hammer grip, maintains palms facing each other. Think of hammer curls, or front delt raises with thumbs leading the way. The overhand grip keeps thumbs facing one another. Your standard incline barbell bench press uses an overhand grip. Reverse/underhand grip is just the opposite, and keeps the pinkies facing one another. These are great for rows, curls, chin-ups, triceps cable extensions and plenty more that I will discuss later.

Each grip variation serves a unique purpose, and you will quickly notice how even a subtle, 90-degree wrist rotation can considerably alter both the strength and the focal point of a contraction. Let's take single-arm cable rows, for example. I might start with hammer grip for about seventeen reps. After two or three sets, I might switch to reverse grip, recruiting more of my lower back. If I can get seventeen on hammer grip, I'm lucky to get fourteen or so with reverse. An even greater drop in strength occurs with an overhand cable row, since your elbow flares out to the side, calling on your upper back, rear delts, and traps to carry the load. You just performed the same exercise in three distinct ways, targeting three different sections of your back simply by rotating your wrist.

As a point of clarity, this change in strength plays no roll in how effective one grip is over another at producing a quality physique; it merely highlights the diversity of the modes in which a single muscle group can contract.

A creative way to take advantage of this strength difference is a mock drop set, where instead of reducing the weight upon reaching failure, you simply switch to a stronger grip to add a few more repetitions and extend the burn. DB shoulder press provides a great opportunity for one of these mock drop sets because of the fact that the lift becomes significantly stronger as the user rotates grips. Start with reverse, as this is the weakest. Once you reach or approach failure, keep the set going by seamlessly switching to the somewhat stronger hammer grip. Continue with this wrist position until you can no longer perform quality reps, and then immediately move into the even stronger overhand DB press. The burn from one of these mock drop sets could most aptly be compared to being hosed down with military-grade napalm after streaking through a field of holly bushes.

Not only should you change grips between sets and reps like this, you should also be rotating during a rep itself. More times than not, I'll rotate my grip *throughout* a single motion, if that particular exercise allows it. With front delt raises, I may have a hammer grip at the starting point, and throughout the squeeze, I might rotate clockwise, ending with an underhand grip at the peak. I may even switch from reverse grip to overhand grip, repeating the mirror image of the movement during the eccentric phase. Several lifts allow room for some in-rep wrist rotation, and I describe each of these in the later sections.

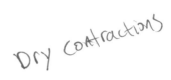
Dry Contractions

Functional Flexing

Now comes arguably the most underutilized strategy in the every-day gym goer: the post-set isometric hold, also referred to as the dry contraction. This involves contracting the muscle you just finished a set with at maximum effort for around ten seconds, without the use of weights. Think this as a way of finishing off the last bit of life your muscles thought they had left. After a good set on decline chest flies, squeeze your palms together about two feet in front of you, right at nipple height. Squeeze like you're trying to fuse your hands into one. If you do it right, your chest will likely cramp up. You may even go to your knees. Good. In order to grow, you must thoroughly eviscerate your muscle fibers. After a set of skull-crushers, lock out your elbows past 180 degrees until your triceps break out into a full-blown spasm. Following a set of dumbbell military press, grab just under your glutes and try to pull your hands clean through your legs until your delts are all but audibly pleading for mercy (You can also press the backs of your hands against the sides of an empty doorframe to target your delts).

Apply this technique to all body parts, repeating four to five times near the end of each workout. The cramping will prematurely exhaust what you have left in the tank, so be sure to get the bulk of your work in be-fore beginning these dry contractions. Executing these consistently will create a much more hardened look while significantly improving your mind-muscle connection. You wouldn't believe how many professional bodybuilders only spend about 30-40 minutes lifting weights, and use the rest of their time posing and performing isometric holds.

You will look utterly deranged as you perform dry contractions. People will slander you. Women will avoid you as if you've tattooed "I have Ebola" in Times New Roman across your forehead. To hell with them. Wanna know what's worse than looking deranged? Looking exactly how you looked three years ago. Swallow your pride and make some progress.

Another way to integrate some functional flexing is through a technique called pulsing. Due to its more advanced nature, proper pulsing requires a fairly advanced mind-muscle connection, so don't be surprised if you're not as fluid with it on your first few attempts. Once you become more comfortable with the concepts discussed so far, though, this is an extremely useful practice that can etch out the fine details and separation within muscle groups that you so desperately crave.

Pulsing involves cutting the full range of motion in two and performing only the upper half of the movement. Thus, the pulsing range of motion spans from the fully flexed position to about halfway back to the starting point. For leg extensions, you should squeeze up to full flex with a light to moderate weight and hold for a moment. Surrender slowly, just as you normally would, only instead of returning to the stretch position, squeeze your quads back up to full flex once you get about halfway down. Using a controlled, rhythmic bounce, keep yourself in this zone of contraction for as long as you can. Every fifth rep or so, hold the squeeze at the top for a few seconds before pulsing some more. Repeat this pattern until you begin to hallucinate, and then apply it to any and every conceivable bodybuilding exercise.

I do not have the words to properly express the wonders that pulsing has done for my physique. It can be applied to every muscle group humans possess, and to date, I have found no more superior practice at chiseling out razor-sharp cuts than that of pulsing. Use these during the last two sets of each movement during your session, perhaps even at the end of a drop set, and you will soon understand where I am coming from.

Ripping Up Routines

In lieu of giving you a set-in-stone lifting program, I have provided a database with some of my favorite exercises and tips for each body part. I do this to emphasize the freedom you should experience with your training. One of the facets of bodybuilding I love so much is that no two workouts have to be the same. Some chest days, I may do twelve separate movements over the course of an hour. Others, I may stick with just two. I might do four distinct supersets on a shoulders/biceps day, and four completely different ones the next. The objective is not to create a mundane, repeatable pattern; the objective is to exert yourself so completely, and to exhaust your muscle fibers so extensively, that your body is *forced* to grow.

That being said, my most commonly followed weekly pattern is as follows: chest, back/triceps, shoulders/biceps, legs, arms, cardio/agility, and then a rest day. Other weeks I may combine chest with back, or legs with biceps, or give an entire day to triceps. I may even do a push/pull/ legs or upper/lower body split for a few weeks. I double up on arms and shoulders most weeks, simply because that's how I want to shape my physique. This is your body. You, and you alone, are in charge of it.] ✳ Treat it as your canvas.

We wear our work

I start each workout with about five minutes of jump rope/elliptical/lunges/A-C skipping, etc. Anything to get my blood moving and my heart rate increased will do. More often than not, I pick one Olympic/powerlifting movement per day, such as military press or back squat, to work on increasing my strength. Starting the majority of my workouts this way has worked best for me over the years, and allows me to train as heavy as possible while my muscles are still fresh. Think of this as the functional section of the workout, with the rest of it focused solely on hypertrophy and aesthetics. Always, always, always start incredibly light, perhaps even with just a bar. Feel the contraction. Watch your form in the mirror. Listen to your body. After a gradual crescendo of three to five weight increases, I perform four to six working sets of 80–95 percent of my max, with no more than a minute of rest in between. After completing these sets, I spend the rest of my time purely bodybuilding, which requires than I shift my mindset from *explosion* to *contraction*.

Generally speaking, I randomly pick four to ten exercises among the lists corresponding to that particular day. The majority of this time is spent engulfed in a near-failure antagonist superset, as I incorporate pulsing, drop sets, grip variations, and dry contractions into the superset itself. With each rep, I internally repeat the mantra "squeeze, surrender, stretch," as I try to make the weight feel as heavy as possible. Implementing these concepts is what is going to transform your physique. Above all else, you must always remember that reducing rest periods is vital to taking full advantage of your limited gym time.

The only way that your five to six hours a week in the gym are going to bring the body of your dreams to fruition is if every last second is accounted for, and every last rep performed with an unbridled intensity. "Time under tension" is a near-ubiquitous concept in the bodybuilding world, and is all about maximizing the proportion of your workout in which your muscles are actually contracting. You should be filling each precious minute in the gym with so much work that you have to bring a water bottle from home because YOU CAN'T EVEN AFFORD TO

SPEND SEVENTEEN SECONDS WALKING TO THE FOUNTAIN! Researchers at the University of Sydney in Australia helped solidify this concept with an experiment performed over two decades ago. Subjects were assigned to either a "rest" group or a "no rest" group. After a six-week training program and with careful consideration to control for variables, the "no rest" group saw a 56 percent increase in dynamic strength, as opposed to a 41 percent increase in the "rest" group (Rooney et al. 1994). If this doesn't violently ram home my point then I don't know what will.

To put things into perspective, consider the fact that a year has but fifty-two weeks. If you spend the standard twenty weeks losing fat (and therefore adding marginal or zero muscle), then you have only thrity-two weeks to grow. Thirty-two weeks means hitting each body part thirty-two times, assuming not one hitch in your schedule. This should ignite a fire under you and illustrate how categorically imperative it is that you wholly exhaust yourself during each of these sessions.

Chest:

Core movements:
> Flat Bench [A] – DB/BB
> Incline Bench [B] – DB/BB
> Decline Bench [C] – DB [D]/BB

Supplementary movements:
> DB Flies [E] – Flat/Incline/Decline
> Around-the-World-DB Flies [F]
> Hammer-Strength Side Press [G]
> Cable Flies [H] – Incline/Standard/Decline
> Pec-Deck Flies
> Dips
> Push-ups

A. Some prefer to wrap the thumb around the bar, while some prefer the "suicide grip" with the thumb underneath. I am a suicide gripper, but it is mostly up to personal preference. Hand spacing on barbell press varies from lifter to lifter as well. I generally go about a hand's length outside of shoulder width, as this creates a broader chest, but others prefer to use a narrower grip to recruit more triceps. Experiment with it and shake things up from week to week to fully develop the entire pectoralis muscle. With light-weight, high-rep sets of flat bench-press, you can create a slight variation by lifting your feet off the floor and extending your legs past the edge of the bench to force your body to use its stabilizing muscles, which are much more difficult to isolate.

B. Contract your abs throughout the entire set. This will keep your lower back flush to the bench, subsequently targeting more of the upper chest, or pectoralis minor. Arching your back is cheating, and will delay your progress.

C. If your gym doesn't have a one-piece decline bench press, you can set up a lone decline bench inside the Smith machine. The same goes for incline. However, anyone using the Smith machine for flat bench press should be euthanized by the federal government.

D. With DB press of any incline, you can get another inch or two of depth in your eccentric phase, since your chest is not blocking the weight. Use this added range of motion to exaggerate the stretch. Remember, the weight should dominate you in this position. At the top of the squeeze, the weights should be touching, meaning that your hands, unlike so with a barbell, become closer together throughout the squeeze and farther apart throughout the surrender. Overhand and hammer grips should be used in equal proportion.

E. Exaggerate the stretch even more so with DB flies. During the concentric phase, move like you're wrapping your arms around a giant Redwood tree. At the top, pretend that a pencil has been laid along your sternum, and try to crush it with your pecs. To help with this, think about pushing your elbows together instead of your hands. Flies are also great for mid-rep wrist rotations. Experiment with lighter weight and see which ones you like best before increasing the weight.

F. Never go above 20–25 pounds. Place the bench at about 30 degrees of incline and completely extend your arms along the same path as your body, holding the dumbbells in an overhand grip. Maintaining a slight elbow bend, create as large of a circle as you can with your hands. At the bottom, you will be in a reverse grip. From here, use your chest to move the weights another eight to twelve inches perpendicular to your body, and then follow the same path in reverse to bring the weights back overhead.

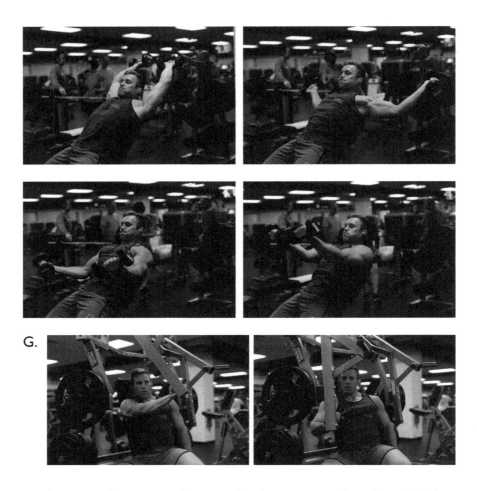

G.

H. Increase the range of motion by five or six inches from DB flies by crossing the hands over top of one another at the end of the squeeze. You will instantly notice the difference in the intensity of contraction. Move the cable position to different heights to target the lower, middle, and upper parts of the chest.

*Remember to do your isometric holds three to five times near the end of your workout, for at least ten seconds each time. Some even place 2.5 or 5-pound barbells in each palm to force themselves to squeeze harder. Experiment with and without weights.

*Your chest fatigues much faster than other body parts, so always have a spotter when supersetting with barbells, as they have been known to crush tracheas.

*Utilize drop sets. One of my favorites is loading five 25-pound plates on each side of a barbell. With a spotter behind me, I will burn out six times back to back, removing a plate after each occurrence, until I am left with only the bar. If 25s are too much, use 10s or 5s.

*"40 Cal's" are a great chest building drill that almost mimics pulsing. These can be performed with DBs or BBs, and any degree of incline/ decline. In a single set, perform ten reps with the bottom third of the motion, ten with the middle third, ten with the top third, and ten with the full range of motion.

*Limit rest periods.

*Squeeze, surrender, stretch.

Back:

Core Movements:
Deadlift [A]
Pull-up [B]
Pull-down [C]
Single-Arm Row [D] – DB/KB
Bent-Over Row [E] – BB/DB (double-arm)/Smith machine
Cable Row – Squatted/seated, double/single arm
T-Bar Row

Supplementary Movements:
Cable Pullover [F]
Romanian Deadlift [G]
Incline Bench Row [H]
Hammer-Strength Row
Superman
Back-Extension
Assisted Pull-up
Rack Pulls [I]
Inverted Rows [J]
Dumbbell Pullovers [K]

A. Focus on contracting your rear traps throughout the movement. This helps to keep your back straight and avoid injuries. The bar should be kept as close to your shins as possible during the concentric phase. Professional powerlifters often wear shin pads to protect against scraping, which should illustrate for you the necessary proximity of the bar and their legs. Keep your feet shoulder width and your grip a hand's length outside of shoulder width. A common mistake I see is guys making the top of the motion a relaxed position. The very top of the deadlift should the most uncomfortable position of the entire movement, as every muscle in your posterior chain should be absolutely torqued beyond comprehension. Your rear delts, traps, lats, rhomboids, erector spinae, hamstrings, glutes, and calves should all be contracting simultaneously.

B. At LEAST fifty every single back day, even if some need to be on the assisted pull-up machine. Even with the assist, pull-ups recruit significantly more muscle than pull-downs. Work on narrow, shoulder width, and wide grip, as well as an overhand, hammer, and reverse grip, while focusing on pulling from your *elbows*.

C. Just like with pull-ups, pull from your elbows and work with all styles of grip. Some days, I might do two sets of wide overhand, two wide hammer, two wide reverse, and then repeat with shoulder-width and narrow grips. Other days I may spend the whole session with a hammer grip. Mix it up as you wish.

D. With a hammer or reverse grip, think about pulling your pinky to your hip with your elbow. With an overhand grip, think about flaring your elbow outward so that it's perpendicular to your torso (requires much lighter weight). When performing any style of a row, the start of the contraction MUST be focused at the scapulae. This will minimize bicep involvement and force your lats, teres, and rhomboids to do the work.

E. Use your hip as a hinge, bending forward slightly and keeping the torso straight. DO NOT bring your chest to the bar; bring the bar to your chest. Again, work with all grip widths and wrist rotations, contracting first at the scapulae.

F. Set the cable system to its highest point with a rope or flat bar/ EZ Curl attachment. Bend 45–60 degrees at the waist so that as you grab the cable attachment, your lats are fully stretched. Keep your elbows extended and use your lats to bring your hands to your quads. You may incorporate a slight hip thrust near the end to facilitate the motion.

G. Straight-leg deadlift with light-moderate weight. Remember to tighten every part of your posterior chain at the top of the movement, just as with a regular deadlift.

H. Lie prone on an incline bench with a dumbbell in each hand. Use gravity and the support of the bench to help intensify the stretch, and row just as you normally would.

I. Think of doing the top half of a deadlift. Place the weight on knee-high safety bars in the squat rack and roll the shoulders back as you contract to full extension.

J. Place a barbell on mid-thigh height safety bars in a squat rack (or Smith machine). Lie supine under the bar, and, engaging your core so as to keep the body erect, pull yourself up so that your nipple line makes contact with the bar.

K.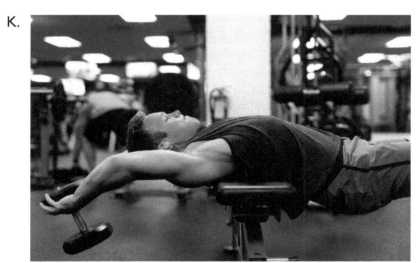

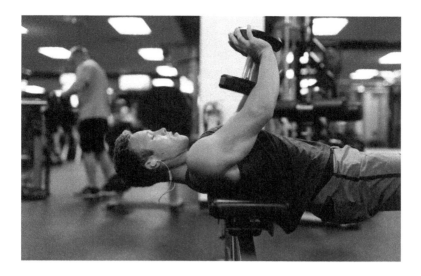

*Back is the easiest body part to cheat reps, which is why most guys' backs are far less developed than the rest of their physique. By keeping your back locked in position during rows and pulldowns, and by using controllable weights, you can avoid this.

*Superset a row with a pull-down/pullover, or a back exercise with a triceps movement to better utilize your time.

*Drop set everything.

*Use lat spreads and back/double-bicep poses for your isometric holds.

*Limit rest periods.

*Squeeze, surrender, stretch.

Biceps:

Standing Curl – DB/BB/KB/EZ Bar/Cable
Seated/Incline-Bench Curl – DB/KB
Preacher Curl – DB/BB/KB/EZ Bar/Cable
    -Spider Curl Variation [A]
Squatted Cable Preacher Curl [B]
Pull/Chin-Up
Zottman DB curl [C]
Seated DB Concentration Curl [D]
Bent-over Single-Arm Cable Curl [E]
Overhead Cable Curl [F]
Lying Cable Curl [G]
Hyper-Extended Cable Curl [H]
"Hanging" Curl [I] – DB/EZ Bar/Fixed Bar

A. Spider curls are preacher curls with the head ducked and the hands finishing above the skull. These are best with an EZ bar, and even better performed if your gym has a preacher setup that allows you to face opposite the intended direction so that at the starting position, your arms are perpendicular to the ground.

B. Place any bar or pair of single handles on the lowest rung of the cable machine and take three big steps back. Squat all the way down, support your elbows with your knees, and extend your arms fully with the weight in hand. As you squeeze, press the elbows down on the knees to provide more leverage.

C. Begin with a hammer grip and arms hanging. With one arm, and keeping your elbow locked onto your rib cage, rotate your palm forward and begin to curl in an outward direction as pictured. Think of moving your hand in a circular motion in front of your body. At the top of the circle, your wrist will be in hammer grip just in front of your shoulder. Continue the circle by crossing the sternum in an overhand grip, and return to the starting position.

This movement is all about fluidity, so grab a light weight and feel a sort of rolling contraction along the entirety of the bicep. After you get the hang of it, try both arms at once, keeping them in perpetual motion so that when one hand is at the top of its circle, the other hand is at its bottom.

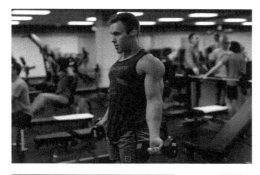

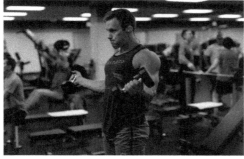

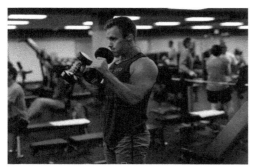

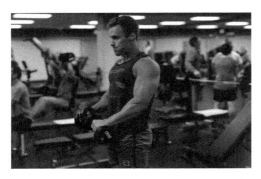

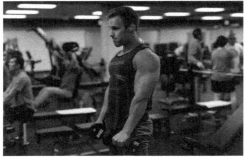

D. Sit on the edge of a bench and lean forward with legs spread. Use the inside of the leg as an anchor for the elbow, just proximal to the knee, so that the arm hangs perpendicular to the ground at the stretch position.

E.

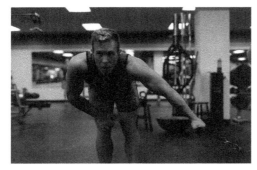

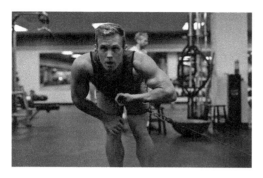

F.

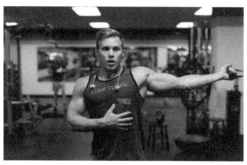

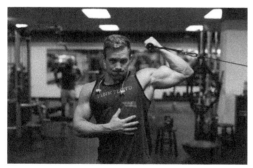

G. Place a clean mat on the floor beside the cable system. Attach any handle you wish to use on the bottom rung of the system. Grab the handle and lie supine on the mat so that the elbows are 180 degrees and curl as normal.

H.

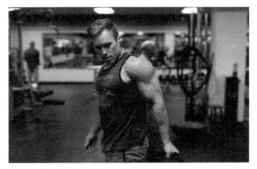

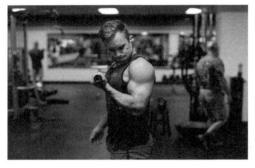

I.

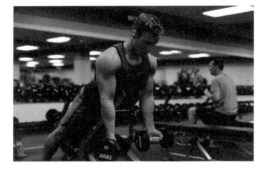

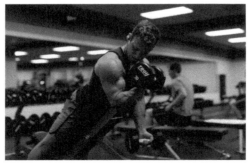

*Anything that can be done with a bar should be done with varying grip widths and anything with a DB/KB/single-arm handle should be done with varying wrist rotations.

*All cable curl variations should be done with any and all attachments, both single and double-arm, including the ropes for cable hammer curls.

*Superset with any triceps, chest, legs or shoulder exercise.

*Drop set everything.

*Isometric holds.

*Limit rest periods.

*Squeeze, surrender, stretch.

Triceps:

Overhead Extension [A] – DB/EZ Bar/Cable
      Standing/Seated/Incline Bench
      Single/Double-Arm
Front-Facing Cable Extension [B]
Skull Crushers [C] – DB/EZ Bar
      Flat/Incline Bench
Bench Dips [D]
Close-Grip Press [E] – BB/DB/EZ Bar [F]
      Flat/Incline Bench
JM Press [G]
      Flat/Incline Bench
Lying Triceps Extension [H] – DB/EZ Bar
      Flat/Incline Bench
Tate Press [I]
Triceps Kickback [J] – DB/KB/Cable [K]
Reverse-Grip Press – BB/DB [L]

A. Allow gravity to enhance the stretch. Let the weight take your hands farther down your back than you ever dreamed possible. You should feel the stretch all the way from your armpits to your elbows. When using the cables, set the apparatus to the bottom of the slide and attach the ropes or two single handles. You can either perform these standing with feet in a runner's stance, or sitting on an incline bench.

B. Use any and all cable attachments and wrist rotations. Lean forward at the waist and use your body weight to assist you with additional reps once you reach failure. You can markedly intensify your lockout contraction by pointing your knuckles to the floor with each rep.

C. Keep the upper half of your arm completely locked, only moving at the elbow joint. With an overhand, underhand, or hammer grip, bring the weight right to the bridge of the nose (EZ Bar) or beside the ears (DBs).

D.

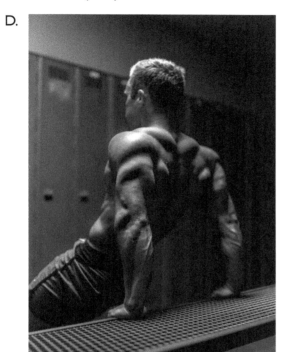

E. Keep hands shoulder-width apart and elbows tucked against your rib cage. Really emphasize your mind-muscle connection to engage the triceps and not the pectoralis. Lighter weight helps with this.

F. These are great for adding extra reps to the end of a set of skull-crushers or lying triceps extension, because it is a much stronger movement, meaning that you can create a mock drop set without even changing position.

G. Think of JM press as a close grip press that brings the bar to your neck instead of your nipple line. Place a flat bench inside of a Smith machine, and adjust your body position so that the bar is directly in line with your neck. With arms shoulder width and elbows tucked, bring the bar down slowly to just below the chin, and push your elbows to the ceiling to amplify the stretch. Press to full extension and repeat.

H. Treat these exactly like skull-crushers, except for the fact that you are bringing the weight overhead and not to the bridge of your nose.

I. Grab a moderate weight dumbbell in each hand and lie on an incline or flat bench. Start with the weights overhead in an overhand grip with elbows locked. Slowly lower both hands down so that the thumb side of the dumbbell lies flat on the chest in the stretch position, and then use the triceps to press the weights back overhead.

J. LIGHT WEIGHT!!!!!!! I routinely see kids half my size doing kickbacks with triple the weight I use. For dumbbells, I tend to stick with 10–15 pounds, so do not feel weird about using 5s. Remember, leave your ego at the door. Bend over at the waist and bring the weight up to your hip, just as you would for a single-arm row. Lock the upper arm in place, and begin to lock out the elbow joint. At the top of the squeeze, flex your wrist along the same plane in such a way that brings the pinky closer to the sides of the wrist. This will enhance the contraction significantly.

K. Use the single handle for reverse grip kickbacks. You may also use no attachment, instead grabbing hold of the hook at the end of the cable.

L. Treat this as a normal BB/DB bench press, but with a reverse grip. For this to work properly, you MUST isolate the triceps, taking the chest out of the equation as much as possible.

*Triceps have some of the toughest fascia in the body, so your squeeze and stretch must be taken to a new level in this section.

*Superset with any biceps, back, or leg exercise.

*Drop set everything.

*Isometric holds.

*Limit rest periods.

*Squeeze, surrender, stretch.

Shoulders

Presses:
>   Military Press – BB/DB/KB/Smith/Hammer Strength
>   >   Seated/Standing
>   >   Single/Double-Arm
>
>   Arnold Press [A]
>   Bradford Press [B]
>   Handstand Pushups

Front Delts:
>   Front Raises [C] – DB/KB/EZ Bar/Cable/Fixed Bar
>   >   Seated/Standing
>   >   Single/Double-Arm
>   Steering Wheels [D]
>   Plate Punches [E]
>   Reverse Grip EZ Bar Press

Lateral Delts:
>   Lateral Raises [F] – DB/KB/Cable/Fixed Bar
>   >   Straight-Arm
>   >   >   Flexed-Arm
>   >   >   Behind-the-back
>   >   Leaning [G]
>   Shoulder Taps [H]
>   DB Salt Pours [I]
>   Sword Pulls [J]
>   One-Arm Static Holds [K]

Rear Delts:
>   Reverse Flies [L] – DB/KB/Cable/Pec Deck
>   Face Pulls [M]
>   Rear Delt Row [N]

Y's/T's/W's ᵒ
"Get Off Me's" ᴾ

Traps:
Shrug – BB/DB/KB/Cable/Smith
High Pull – BB/DB/KB/Cable/Smith
Power Clean
Hang Clean
Snatch

A. Perform a normal DB press, but upon reaching the starting position in overhand grip, rotate the shoulders so as to bring the weights in front of the chin in a reverse grip. Feel the stretch of the front deltoid, and then rotate back to overhand grip beside the head, and press upward once more. Be advised, you will need much lighter weight when using an Arnold Press than you will during a standard DB military press.

B. Same as BB Military Press, only a single rep is counted as starting behind the head, pressing to full extension, returning to front of face, pressing again to full extension, and returning to behind the head.

C. Great for experimenting with wrist rotations, both intra-set and intra-rep. Use full range of motion, which is from a dead hang to straight overhead. NO ROCKING. The only muscle on your body that should contract (besides forearms to hold the weight) is your front deltoid.

D. Use a 10–25 pound BB weight as a steering wheel, holding at nine and three o'clock. With arms fully extended and knees slightly flexed, rotate the "steering wheel" back and forth until you reach the point of failure.

E. Grab a 10–45 pound BB weight, holding just as with steering wheels. Start with the weight held against your chest, and "punch" both arms forward with each rep.

F. Use your mind-muscle connection to target your shoulder caps and not your traps. To help with this, try cocking your wrists back like you're revving a motorcycle engine. Use all wrist rotations, incline-bench degrees, cable connections, hand paths, anything to create a different angle.

G. Grab ahold of a weight tree, squat rack, cross-over machine, or anything that can support your body weight, as you lean several degrees to the side. With a weight in the hanging arm, perform these more isolated lateral raises.

H. Get into handstand pushup position, but instead of pushing, alternate each hand in tapping the opposing shoulder. Obviously, a single arm will be supporting the entire bodyweight for the majority of this exercise, so do try and avoid severing your spinal cord.

I. In this lateral raise variation, hold a lighter DB in each hand directly in front of you with elbows bent 90 degrees. Pretend the DB is a jar of salt. Lock the wrists and elbows in place throughout the movement as you "pour the salt" out of the jars. Your hands should create a C that tops out at forehead height.

J.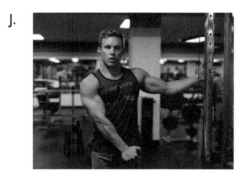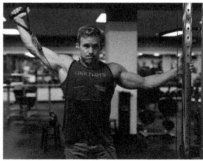

K. Perform a standard single-arm lateral delt raise while the opposite arm holds a 5–15 pound weight in the lateral raise squeeze position throughout the set.

L. LIGHT WEIGHT!!!!!! Rear delts are extremely weak muscles, but can make monumental differences in your overall shoulder development. Use hammer and overhand grips with high elbow angles as you bend at the waist or lie prone on a low-incline bench. Be careful not to use your rhomboids or traps.

M. Place a ropes connection on the seated cable row, and grab so that the backs of your hands are facing each other. Using a light weight, pull with the rear delts to bring the apex of the rope to the bridge of your nose.

N. Place a very light weight (Less than 95 pounds) on a BB and bend 90 degrees at the waist. Using ONLY your rear delts, pull the bar to your chin.

O.

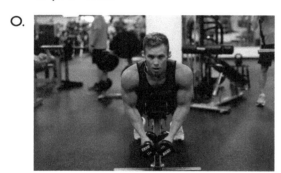

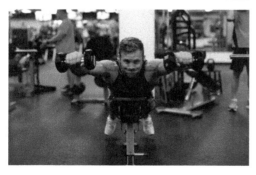

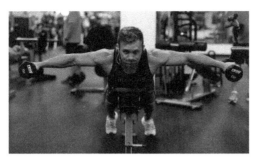

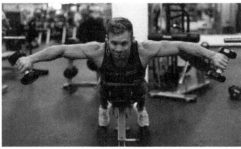

P.   Place a single handle attachment on the bottom rung of the cable system. Face the cables and turn 90 degrees in either direction so that the handle is beside you. Bend at the waist, grab the handle with the far hand, and use the rear delts to pull the elbow across the body until your hand is adjacent to the ipsilateral shoulder. The name stems from the idea of elbowing a would-be attacker standing behind you.

*Superset any two movements from different shoulder subcategories (press, lateral, front, rear, traps), or any shoulder movement with a back, leg, or biceps movement.

*Drop set everything.

*Isometric holds.

*Limit rest periods.

*Squeeze, surrender, stretch.

Legs:

BB Back Squat [A]
BB Front Squat [B]
Hack Squat [C]
Leg Press [D]
Weighted Lunge [E]
Bench Lunge [F]
Leg Extensions
Hamstring Curls
Calf Raises [G]
Goblet Squat [H]
Jefferson Squat [I]
Cannon Ball Squat [J]

A. Feet just outside of shoulder width with toes pointed slightly outward. Keep your core tight and your scapulae retracted for the entire set. Sink back with your hips and maintain the bulk of the weight on your heels.

B. If you are not flexible enough to do crossfit-style front squats, you can cross your hands in front of your body and hold the bar on top of your front delts. Emphasize the quads more than the hamstrings with this movement.

C. Place the feet at the top of the foot board to target the hamstrings and place them at the bottom to target the quads. Experiment with toes pointed outward and inward to develop the entire group of leg muscles.

D. Place the feet near the top of the sled to target more of the hamstrings, and place them at the bottom to target the quads. Vary the width of your feet as well as the angle that your toes point, so as to engage each part of the quad equally.

E. Place a weighted barbell over your back as you would with a back squat, or hold a dumbbell in each hand. Engage the core to help balance. Longer strides work more of the hamstrings while shorter strides focus more on the quads.

F. With one foot supported on top of a flat bench, and a dumbbell in each hand, sink forward over the toes of your down foot. Engage the core to help balance.

G. Whether you perform these on a calf raise machine, the leg press sled, or by standing on the edges of two barbell plates with weights in each hand or a barbell on your back, always switch up the angle of your toes between neutral, inward, and outward.

H. Hold a dumbbell or kettlebell directly in front of the chin, supporting with the palms, using the weight as a counterbalance to allow a deeper hip sink.

I. Use a light weight on a barbell and place the bar on the floor, directly between both feet. Keeping one foot on either side of the bar and the center of the bar below your torso, stagger your feet so as to put you into a modified lunge position with the right foot forward. Open the left (rear) foot so that it points perpendicular to the front foot and squat down. With the right hand, grab the bar in an underhand grip in front of the body. With the left hand, grab the bar with an overhand grip behind the body, and then engage your glutes and hamstrings to stand up. Repeat the process with the mirrored foot position.

J. Place a 45-pound BB weight inside the squat rack where your feet should go. With the weight on your back, stand so that your heels are elevated on the weight, toes pointed out, and feet inside shoulder witch.

*Do not neglect your legs!! Not only will your physique look incomplete, but you will miss out on immeasurable amounts of testosterone released from working the largest muscles in the human body, the quads.

*Superset a quad exercise with a hamstring or calf-focused movement, or any leg movement with another body part you wish to target on that day.

*Drop set everything.

*Isometric holds.

*Limit rest periods.

*Squeeze, surrender, stretch.

Cardio

Let's talk about the elephant in the room. And no, I am not referring to a topic we've both been avoiding; I'm talking about you – you're the elephant. It's time to lose some weight, and unless you plan on paying some metrosexual Botox junkie from Los Angeles to suck the fat from your hips through a sterilized Dyson tubo-vac, then cardio is about to become your new best friend. Some of you think that cardio is Spanish for "lift faster" and the other half thinks it's a Nazi-funded plague aimed at depopulating the masses. Allow me to set the record straight.

Thankfully for you, getting lean does not necessitate spending countless hours performing low intensity steady state (LISS) cardio on the cross-trainer. While this certainly will burn fat and retain muscle, and while most top-level professionals utilize this method, there is simply not enough time in the day for normal, working people like you and me to justify that practice. The popularity of high intensity interval training (HIIT) has grown astronomically over the past decade, as people have come to experience not only its time-efficiency, but its breadth of overall health benefits— which far exceed sheer aesthetic enhancements.

HIIT is designed for users to spend several brief stints in a maximal effort state, with the goal of exceeding 80 percent of your peak oxygen uptake (VO_{2peak}), followed by quick recovery periods (Burgomaster et al., 2005). The science behind HIIT is still in the early stages, but the results thus far have been remarkable, specifically with regard to oxygen transport and consumption.

Researchers at the Department of Kinesiology at McMaster University in Ontario found a 15–35 percent increase in muscle oxidative capacity, "assessed using the maximal activity or protein content of mitochondrial enzymes" in moderately active, college-aged men and women after just six HIIT sessions over a two week span (Gibala and McGee, 2008). In layman's terms, this means that HIIT markedly improved a given muscle's ability to utilize the oxygen molecules at its disposal, a critical component for both hypertrophy and overall well-being.

Incredible as this finding may be, it becomes a moot point without a healthy, functioning cardiovascular system to allow adequate *delivery* of these oxygen molecules so they may actually be used. LISS cardio has long been considered the preeminent physical method for improving vascular health. However, a 2008 study at the Ivor Wynne Centre's Department of Kinesiology showed no statistically significant advantage when comparing peripheral artery distensibility between subjects completing six weeks of long endurance training and those engaging in six weeks of HIIT (Rakobowchuk et al. 2008). So, despite spending less than a QUARTER of the time actually exercising, the HIIT group saw roughly the SAME improvement in arterial condition!

Still, do remain ever cognizant of the inverse relationship between time and effort when comparing LISS and HIIT. Cramming the equivalent caloric output of an hour's worth of elliptical training into ten short minutes is no leisurely task, as your fellow gym patrons should quickly notice. If your name has yet to appear on an FBI watch list after a handful of HIIT workouts at your local YMCA, then chances are you need to reevaluate the effort you're bringing to the table. Leading up to pool season, work in two ten-minute HIIT segments per week at the end of your lift, and then another twenty- to thirty-minute segment on a non-lifting day.

Most often, I spend half of my HIIT session rotating between a randomly selected circuit of two to four exercises listed below, as I spend about 60-120 seconds at maximum effort, and 20-30 seconds resting.

KB Swings
Jumping Lunges
Mountain Climbers
Thrusters
Push Press
Wall Balls
Jump Rope
Row Machine
Battle Ropes
Burpees
Box Jumps
Death Drops
Farmer's Carry
Squat Jumps
Ski Erg

I generally utilize Tabata-style sprinting for the second half of my cardio. Developed by Japanese scientist Izumi Tabata, this system involves twenty to thirty seconds of all-out expenditure followed by ten to fifteen seconds rest. This can be done on a treadmill at a speed of ten to twelve and as much incline as you can handle, or sprinting on a track or up a hill. Where you perform these sprints is much less important than the stringency of your counting; ten seconds rest does not mean two minutes. You should be on the verge of projectile vomiting by the end of this onslaught.

Way too many people are afraid to maximally exert themselves at the gym out of fear of what someone they BARELY know may think. You simply have GOT to get over this if you wish to make any progress. I'm not saying that people should be able to hear you moaning from the parking lot, but God forbid you break a sweat and lose your breath from time to time. I for one get jacked up when I see someone pushing the limits, and it unconsciously gives me permission to do the same. Sure, you may look a bit unhinged in the moment, but you're going to look SICK when beach season rolls around.

Abs:

There are dozens of abdominal exercises, and even more opinions on the subject. Some pros never train abs, others train seven days a week. Some only train weighted abs, others stick to body weight. Some avoid oblique work to keep a slimmer profile, while others use rotational exercises to bring out the serratus muscle striations. I can only tell you what has worked for me, which is two ten-minute sessions per week, with a 50/50 split between weighted and bodyweight exercises. Weighted abdominal movements produce some thickness to the muscles, a crucial aspect for creating the deep cuts that bring your six-pack to life. Some of you may flinch at that notion, as you want to keep a slender build, but understand that abs don't go from flat to bulky overnight. They need a little bit of mass to show definition, and that takes time. Also, "bulky abs" is just a euphemism for a poor diet and lack of cardio.

The biggest key is applying the squeeze, surrender, stretch technique to each and every rep in the gym. Abs recover quickly, so in order to force improvement, your entire session must be agonizing. The number of sit-ups, or leg raises, or L-sits, or scissor kicks you perform is irrelevant; lengthening the TIME you spend in the burn is the goal. Even as your form begins to fade and your consciousness starts slipping into oblivion, stay with the burn. Most gyms come equipped with a defibrillator, so you have a pretty decent shot of being revived should your heart stop beating. If not, I can confidently say that your death will serve the grand purpose of strengthening the ever-weakening gene pool plaguing this planet.

Another way to bring out some abdominal definition is through vacuuming. No, I'm not talking about erasing the evidence of that handful of Oreos you choked down at 3 a.m. when you thought I wasn't watching, I'm referring to an exercise. With an empty stomach, take a deep breath in and expand your belly. As you empty your lungs, suck your stomach in as hard as you can, trying to touch your belly button to your spinal cord. Hold this position with the lungs empty for five to ten seconds before releasing tension, taking a breath, and repeating for fifteen reps two to three times per week. Vacuuming recruits the transverse abdominal muscles, which are difficult to isolate, but serve to slim the waist line and keep everything nice and tight. It will be painful at first, and you may not be able to hold for the entire set, but stick with it and you will develop quickly.

Sample 12-Week Program

Use this as a general framework for something I would loosely follow over a three-month period. I say loosely because my workouts are MY time. If I get three sets into a shoulder day and suddenly decide that I would be much happier blasting my biceps into oblivion, then that is exactly what I am going to do. Feel free to swap out whole sections for something completely different, or adjust the rep ranges to fit your preference. If you get in the groove on back squats one day and want to spend your entire session there, then by all means, GET AFTER IT! Do not allow yourself to be shackled by the strictures of a defined exercise regimen. *Take control of your life!*

Note that for each month-long phase, I have only included a single week of exercises. This is because, for the rest of the month, I want you to create your own routine based on the given week's layout. For example, take a look at Phase 1's Wednesday workout. Maybe for week 2 you swap out military press for Arnold press, or front delt raises for steering wheels, or shrugs for hang cleans. This is YOUR body and YOUR time, so do with it as you like. Hopefully this framework will give you a general idea of how to attack the gym and build a schedule that fits your needs.

The first phase of this example places emphasis on hypertrophy and perfecting your mind-muscle connection with lighter weights. "Squeeze, surrender, stretch" should be your sole focus in the gym during these four weeks. I have provided a WIDE target rep range for each set to underscore that reaching exhaustion is the ultimate goal. Adjust weights between sets so as to provide the right amount for that particular range, but NEVER cut a set short just because you've reached a given number of reps. Also, do not forget to implement your isometric holds, pulsing, grip variations, and all of the concepts we have covered thus far.

Phase two moves into heavier weight and lower reps to improve your strength with your newly-improved form. This will require you to adjust to a more explosive mindset and deviate from pure hypertrophy for a bit. You may not be as sore during this month, as strength training targets the central nervous system more so than the actual muscle, but I assure you that your muscles will be stimulated appropriately. This phase will also lower your tolerance to the high-rep contraction-focused style lifting of phase one, which will help to reaccelerate your progress upon starting over. The rep ranges are much lower, but they are still designed for you to be around the point of exhaustion by the end of each set, so increase the weight until you cannot exceed the given ranges.

The final month is a combination of the previous two, in which you will be utilizing a Push/Pull/Legs split. Altering your routines in this manner forces your body to constantly adapt to changing stimuli, ensuring that maximal stress is always being applied and fostering an environment that blasts through plateaus.

PHASE I (weeks 1-4)

Monday: Chest/Biceps

Active Warm-up	5 Min.
Push-up	3 x 20-40

Superset <

Chin-up	50 Total
Incline DB Bench Press	5 x 15-25

Superset <

Incline DB Hanging Curl	5 x 15-30
Flat BB Bench Press	4 Triple Drops

Super drop <

Squatted Cable Preacher Curl	4 Double Drops
Around-The-World Fly	3 x 10-15

Superset <

Hammer Curl	3 Triple Drops
Weighted Ab Circuit	8 Min.

Tuesday: Back/Triceps

Active Warm-up	5 Min.
Wide-Grip Pull-up	3 x Failure

Superset <

Dips	3 x Failure
T-Bar Row	4 x 15-20

Superset <

Overhead DB Extension	4 x Failure
Neutral/Narrow-Grip Pulldown	3 Double Drops

Superset <

Reverse-Grip Cable Extension	3 Triple Drops
Overhand Smith Machine Row	3 x 12-25

Superset <

JM Press	3 x Failure
RDL	3 x 15-20

Superset <

	DB Kick-back	3 x Failure
	HIIT circuit	10 Min.

Wednesday: Shoulders/Traps

	Active Warm-Up:	5 Min.
	Standing Military Press	5 x 10-20

Superset <

	DB Rear Delt Fly	5 x 10-15
	Reverse-Grip EZ-Bar Press	4 x 20-30

Superset <

	DB Lateral Raise	4 x 12-20
	Cable Sword Pull	3 Double Drops

Super Drop <

	Neutral-Grip Front Raise	3 Double Drops
	EZ-Bar High Pull	3 x 15-25

Superset <

	Smith Machine Shrug	3 x Failure
	Bodyweight Ab Circuit	8 Min.

Thursday: Arms

	Active Warm-up:	5 Min.
	Seated EZ-Bar Preacher Curl	4 x 8-30

Superset <

	Incline EZ-Bar Skull Crusher	4 x 10-20
	Overhead Cable Curl	3 x Failure

Superset <

	Cable Ropes Extension	3 Double Drops
	Standing BB Curl	4 x 20

Superset <

Bench Dip	4 x 10-15
Incline Bench KB Curl	1 Triple Drop
Incline DB Overhead Extension	1 x Failure

Triple set<

Incline Tate Press (Same DBs^)	1 x Failure

Triple set cont. <

Incline Rvrs.-Grip Press (Same DBs)	1x Failure
HIIT Circuit	10 Min.

Friday: Legs

Active Warm-up	5 Min.
Leg Extension	3 x 10-20

Superset <

Hamstring Curl	3 x 8-15
Cannonball Squat	6 x 8-20

Superset <

Calf Raises	6 x 20-30
Back Squat	3 Double Drops
Weighted Lunge	3 x 15-20

Superset <

Goblet Squat	3 x 10-15
Weighted Ab Circuit	8 Min.

Saturday: Agility/Cardio

Active Warm-up	5 Min
HIIT Circuit w/ Tabata Sprints	20-30 Min.
Light-Moderate Jog	3-5 Miles

Sunday: Stretch/Recover

PHASE II (Weeks 5-8)

Monday: Legs

Active Warm-up	5 Min.
BB Back Squat	6 x 3
	2 x 5
Leg Press	6 x 5
Single-Leg Extension	5 x 8
Smith Machine Calf Raise	3 x 10
Weighted Ab Circuit	8 Min.

Tuesday: Back

Active Warm-up	5 Min.
BB Deadlift	8 x 4
V-Bar Cable Row	6 x 8
Neutral/Wide Grip Pulldown	6 x 6
Hammer-Grip DB Row	5 x 8
Pull-up	50 Total
HIIT Circuit	10 Min.

Wednesday: Chest

Active Warm-up	5 Min.
BB Incline Bench Press	2 x 2
	3 x 5
DB Flat Bench Press	2 x 3
	4 x 6
Decline DB Fly	4 x 12-20

Superset <

Push-up	4 x Failure
Cable Crossover Fly	3 Double Drops
Bodyweight Ab Circuit	

Thursday: Arms

Active Warm-up	5 Min.
Standing BB Curl	6 x 8

Superset <

Rvrs-Grip EZ-Bar Skull Crusher	6 x 5-10
Hanging Spider Curl	4 x 10-14

Superset <

Supine Cls-Grip EZ-Bar Press	4 x 6-12
Seated DB Concentration Curl	4 x 8-12

Superset <

Cable Triceps Kickback	4 x 9-15
HIIT Circuit	8 Min.

Friday: Shoulders

Active Warm-up	5 Min.
Seated Military BB Press	8 x 3
	2 x 1
Leaning Fixed Bar Lateral Raise	5 x 8-10
Hammer-Strength Press	4 x 4-8
Pec-Deck Rear Fly	4 x 10-15
Smith Machine Shrug	5 x 4
Single-Arm Cable Front Raise	4 x 6-12

Weekend: Stretch/Recover

PHASE III (Weeks 9-12)

Monday: Push

Active Warm-up:	5 Min.
Seated DB Press	4 x 10-20
Decline BB Bench Press	5 x 5-12
Standing Lateral Raise	3 Double Drops

Superset <

Close-Grip Flat Bench Press	3 x 8-12
Incline DB Bench Press	4 Single Drops
Steering Wheel	3 x 8-15

Superset <

V-Bar Cable Triceps Extension	5 x 12
Bodyweight Ab Circuit	8 Min.

Tuesday: Pull

Active Warm-up	5 Min.
BB Deadlift	5 x 3-8

Superset <

Standing KB Curl	5 x 10-12
Wide/Reverse-Grip Pulldown	4 Triple Drops

Super Drop <

Cable Pullover	4 Double Drops
Single-Arm Rvrs-Grip DB Row	4 x 5-8
Zottman Curl	4 x 15-20

Superset <

Superman	3 x 20
HIIT Circuit	10-15 Min.

Wednesday: Legs

Active Warm-up	5 Min.
Hack Squat	5 x 10-15
Jefferson Squat	3 x 15-20

Superset <

Leg Extension	3 Triple Drops
Narrow-Stance Leg Press	4 x 10-25

Superset <

Calf Raise on Leg Press Sled	4 x 12-20
Walking Long-Stride Lunge	3 x 40 steps
Weighted Ab Circuit	8 Min.

Thursday: Push

Active Warm-up	5 Min.
Flat BB Bench Press	4 x 8-12
	1 Triple Drop
Seated BB Bradford Press	4 x 15-25

Superset <

Decline Cable Fly	4 Double Drops
DB Salt Pour	4 x 12-15

Superset <

EZ-Bar Overhead Extension	4 x 20-30
Pec-Deck Fly	3 x 12-25

Superset <

Plate Punch	3 x 10-15
Narrow/Ovrhnd-Grip Cable Ext.	2 Quad Drops
HIIT Circuit	10 Min.

Friday: Pull

Active Warm-up	5 Min.
Bent-Over Rvrs-Grip BB Row	5 x 10-15

Superset <

BB Shrug (same weight^)	5 x 15-20
V-Bar Pulldown	4 Double Drops

Superset <

Fixed Bar Rear Delt Row	4 x 12-15

EZ-Bar Reverse-Grip Curl	4 x 8-20
Superset <	
DB RDL	4 x 10-20
Ropes Cable Curl	3 Triple Drops
Superset <	
DB Pullovers	3 x 8-12

Saturday: Legs

Active Warm-up	5 Min.
Back Squat	5 x 8-12
	1 Triple Drop
Bench Lunge	3 x 10-15
Superset <	
Goblet Squat	3 x 12-20
Hip Abductor/Adductor	3 x 20-30
Standing Hamstring Curl	4 x 10-20
HIIT Circuit	10 Min.

Sunday: Stretch/Recover

To The Kitchen!

Before we delve into the realm of nutrition, we must first compre-
hensively shift your attitude regarding food. Until you accept the fact
that food is purely for fuel and not reward, and that what you put into
today's body literally becomes tomorrow's body, you will never see the
results you think you deserve. Lifting is the fun part, but the kitchen is
where the real gains are made.

Vastly more important than being honest with which weights you can
actually handle in the gym is being honest about your diet. There isn't
an algorithm in the known universe that could accurately account for
the number of people who have told me that they just can't seem to
lose weight despite eating nothing but chicken and rice. Really? So
we're just going to gloss over the ungodly amount of Alfredo sauce you
drowned your dinner with last night? So we're going to assume the bag
of Cheetos you inhaled between meals today just evaporated through
your skin? Wow. The search is over, everyone. We have officially found
the only mammal in the history of mankind who can vaporize un-
wanted calories without storing them as fat. What a monumental day
for scientists all over the globe.

Allow me to make myself abundantly clear: the reason you are built like a hot tub of Play-Doh is because your diet is trash. Admit it, learn from it, and fix it.

Being perfect is not the goal, but I think we can all agree that just because you managed to last fifteen minutes on the elliptical at the blistering pace of six miles per hour doesn't mean you've earned yourself a triple scoop of Cold Stone fudge. This is by far the most bewildering pattern I've witnessed over the years. It's like watching a wild orangutan on a National Geographic documentary whose lack of a prefrontal cortex has robbed his ability to piece together a rational string of thoughts. Imagine running a marathon in which all 26.2 miles were ran at a 30 percent uphill gradient. Treating yourself to ice cream after a workout is analogous to reaching the five mile marker of the race and subsequently celebrating by rollerblading back to the starting position. It felt awesome didn't it? I hate you.

Stop being an "I'm trying" guy. "I'm trying" guys are pathetic.

Don't TRY to eat better. F***ing do it.

Don't TRY to stop drinking soda. F***ing stop.

Don't TRY to lose weight. F***ing lose weight.

Changing your diet seems unbearable at first, but only because you've never pushed yourself in this area before. After forcing yourself to suffer for a couple of weeks (poor baby ☹), eating correctly will become second nature. Then, and only then, will you begin making real, measurable progress. It will also improve your skin, your sleep schedule, your poops, and almost everything else that's wrong with that sack of despair you call a body.

That being said, I am well aware that we humans are imperfect beings. You are going to slip up from time to time, and that is totally fine. Like I said, I don't want you missing any concerts or bachelor's weekends just to work on your quad separation in the gym. But, understand that if you spend Saturday and Sunday as a commemorative Chris Farley caricature, then come Monday, you will have to BALANCE THE SCALE! Start earning your debaucherous weekends by being PERFECT during the week.

Earn your weekend

I keep my diet as simple as possible. From September through February, I go through a bulking phase, in which my carb intake is significantly higher. From March through August, I go through a cutting phase, during which I cycle my carbs, waxing, and waning throughout the week.

Bulking Season

My daily diet during bulking generally looks like this:

*5 meals (One of which = 50 g whey protein)
*1g protein per pound of body weight dispersed evenly between meals
*2 full servings of vegetables
*3 servings of fruit
*3,000 mg Krealkalyn (EFX brand)
*3–4 cups of rice or 3–4 large potatoes

My protein source is normally eggs, chicken, or tilapia, as these are the cheapest in bulk, but whatever you like will suffice. You will feel full often, and you will put on weight quickly, especially with the krealkalyn (buffered creatine). If you've always been a skinny guy, do not be afraid of growing a winter coat. Unless you plan on ramming a needle in your glutes every morning, your muscles are simply not going to grow in a single-digit body fat state. Say you want to add ten pounds of lean body mass by the start of next summer. You need to start looking at that ten pounds as your *net* gain. In order to reach this ten pound net gain, you have to set your sights on a *total* weight gain of at least twenty-five pounds.

Trust me, the carb cycling diet will get you ready for summer in plenty of time. My heaviest weight of all time was 221 pounds. I looked like a straight-up tick. My jaw line could have been sponsored by Spalding. I had to sleep on my stomach because, similar to the common cockroach, I was physically incapable of rolling off my back. This was all intentional. After a few months of carb cycling, I had melted away the repulsive, walrus-like blubber that had been insulating my newly generated muscle tissue. I was like a beautiful butterfly bursting free from my cocoon, leaving behind the hideous, foul-smelling caterpillar I once was.

LOL (handwritten margin note)

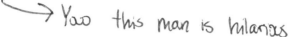
→ Yoo this man is hilarious (handwritten note)

Shredding Season

Carb cycling is certainly under-researched, but the subjective results, based upon fat loss and muscle retention of professional bodybuilders and fitness models, are staggering. There are loads of different patterns one may follow, and I encourage each of you to investigate them for yourself. I have experimented with several of these, and will share with you the one which has worked best for me over the years. Keep in mind that I am generally between 195–215 pounds, so you may need to adjust somewhat to curtail this to your body. I have tried getting people to count macronutrients and calories in the past, but found that adherence quickly becomes an issue with the seemingly never-ending calculations. Carb cycling, on the other hand, minimizes user nuisance and allows for a degree of freedom necessary for a hectic schedule.

>*5 meals (One of which = 50g whey protein)
>*1.5g protein per pound of body weight dispersed evenly
> between meals
>*3 full servings of vegetables
>*2 servings of fruit
>*1,500 mg Krealkalyn

*Brown rice/sweet potato with meals 1–4 as listed below
*Zero added carbs for meal 5—protein and vegetables only

Sat. & Sun.	0
Monday	1/4
Tuesday	1/2
Wed	3/4
Thursday	1
Friday	1

The fractions listed above correspond to the serving of carbs you are to consume with meals 1–4 on that particular day. Think of a full serving as a fist-sized sweet potato or one cup of brown rice. So on Monday, you are to eat a quarter of a sweet potato or a quarter cup of brown rice with each of your first four meals. Tuesday, that amount is doubled, and you are to eat half a serving with meals 1–4. Your carbs are increased throughout the week so that by Thursday and Friday, you are eating a full cup or an entire sweet potato with each of your first four meals. Saturday and Sunday, you are to add no carbs whatsoever, except for vegetables and fruit.

Cutting out carbs entirely is a surefire way to lose weight. The problem is that before long, your muscle stores begin to waste away with the fat. Carb cycling's basic premise is to spend a few days in a zero or low carb state, during which your acutely starving body turns to adipose tissue (fat) as its fuel source. Just before the natural fuel-source conversion from fat to skeletal muscle tissue begins, you provide progressively increasing amounts of glucose so as to regenerate glycogen stores and prevent muscle atrophy without creating a surplus that will be stored as fat. You will be eating a ton of carbs on Thursday and Friday, something that may seem contraindicated for a fat-loss diet. However, this transient excess of calories throws your metabolism into overdrive mode, as it tries to keep up with the increased burden you have introduced. The body will stay in this overdrive mode for the next few days, during which you are significantly reducing your dietary intake. With the metabolism starving for fuel and the stomach providing mere scraps, the body begins digesting fat.

I am not suggesting that carb cycling is the best way to incinerate fat and retain muscle; I am declaring it. Almost every professional bodybuilder and fitness model in the world practices some form of carb cycling. It is the closest thing to a silver bullet that we have found.

You may be thinking that cooking four meals a day is just not possible with your busy schedule. That excuse would be much more plausible had you not spent an hour yesterday afternoon Facebook-stalking that Chloe chick you hooked up with three years ago. What if you multitasked for just fifteen minutes, as you threw a few sliced chicken breasts on two different skillets, cooking rice on the side and microwaving a potato or two at the same time? Suddenly it becomes doable. I am perpetually hurried, and even I can find fifteen minutes to let my food cook on the side while I have a cup of coffee or check the news.

Keep in mind that, while following this diet to a T will produce extraordinary results, you are afforded some flexibility. If you want to get a burger on Friday, count the bun as your full carb serving for that meal and do some extra cardio the next day. If you tend to splurge on the weekends, then shift the days around so that Saturday and Sunday are your high-carb days, and Monday starts back with zero. Do note though, that this weekly layout is specifically designed for you to look your best on Saturdays and Sundays. Monday through Wednesday, your body will be in a depleted state as the glycogen stores you built up have been spent during the zero-carb weekend. Your muscles will appear flat, your definition and strength will be noticeably diminished, and you will struggle mightily to attain even a modest pump in the gym (DO NOT LET YOUR MIND PLAY TRICKS ON YOU—STAY THE COURSE). By Thursday and Friday, your pumps and strength will return like the Prodigal Son, and your muscles will fill out once again.

However, the sheer volume of carbs you will consume is going to bloat your stomach substantially for those two days. By Saturday, you get the best of both worlds; a carbless, flat stomach along with glycogen-filled muscle bellies. Once you get down to about 8 percent body fat, the daily changes in your physique are nothing short of mind-boggling.

You should be weighing yourself first thing Monday morning (or whichever day follows two consecutive 0-carb days) each week to assess your progress. As a rule of thumb, shoot for one to two pounds per week if you want sustainable, healthy weight loss without withering away all the muscle you built thus far. If at six weeks in, you have lost less than six pounds, then adjust your carb cycling as follows:

Sat. & Sun.	0
Monday	1/4
Tuesday	1/4
Wednesday	1/2
Thursday	1/2
Friday	1

Supplements

There are no magic ingredients, so don't buy into the hype of some coked out strip-club owner selling erection pills in a Youtube Ad. A protein supplement is just that: a supplement. Treat it as a substitute for a couple of chicken breasts, and a convenient way to increase your protein intake so as to reach your daily goal. Most brands are virtually identical, so there is no need to break the bank. Get something affordable, low in carbs, and tasty enough to choke down once a day. Optimum Nutrition and MusclePharm are my two favorite brands.

A much more effective supplement at improving one's physique is Kre-Alkalyn. This is a cheap, buffered creatine that, due to its alkaline pH, degrades much more slowly than other forms of creatine in extremely acidic environments, such as the stomach (Golini, 2015). A nonprotein amino acid found naturally in the body, creatine has been among the most widely used performance-enhancing products for decades, as it has been proven time and time again to increase lean body mass, strength, and endurance in athletes of all levels. Its principal metabolic function is to enzymatically combine with a phosphoryl group to form phosphocreatine, which can then be used in the production of cellular fuel (Kreider et al. 2017). Individual cells derive the bulk of their energy from hydrolysis of adenosine triphosphate (ATP), which creates the lower-energy compound adenosine diphosphate (ADP). In the event that ATP reserves are running low, such as in times of intense physical exertion, the phosphoryl group detaches from the creatine molecule, combines with ADP, and forms ATP (Kreider et al. 2017). This additional ATP increases work capacity and thus accelerates progress in all athletic endeavors.

You will also be pleasantly surprised at the size improvements proliferated by Kre-Alkalyn consumption. By considerably escalating the water volume of skeletal muscle cells, creatine has an uncanny ability to effectively and rapidly pack on lean body mass (Hall & Thomas, 2013). Water makes up over 70 percent of muscle composition, so the more volume an individual muscle cell can contain, the larger and fuller its corresponding muscle will appear.

Creatine monohydrate tends to produce very similar results to Kre-Alkalyn with regard to hypertrophy and strength, but is widely known to trouble users with substantial stomach bloating. While most of the evidence in this realm is purely circumstantial, I have yet to hear any similar complaints about Kre-Alkalyn. EFX Brand has worked best for me. Buy it online in pill form and take four per day when bulking or two per day when cutting.

Preworkout drinks are another staple in my regimen, and provide much more benefit than simply a boost in energy. The vasodilation brought about by the L-arginine and niacin allows increased blood flow and, by proxy, increased transport of oxygen to the muscle cells. Beta-alanine is included in most pre-workouts, and once consumed, this non-essential amino acid combines with l-histidine to form carnosine (Artioli et al. 2010). Carnosine then acts as a pH buffer, helping to decrease lactic acid buildup in muscle cells (Helms et al. 2014). With less lactic acid buildup, your muscles will fatigue much later, allowing you to significantly increase their work capacity. After trying dozens of brands, I now prefer C4 Ripped, as it does not have the creatine monohydrate of regular C4 and other formulas. With that shake, I take 500 mg of magnesium for vascular support and I additional gram of L-arginine to dilate the veins even further. You can pick both of these up at any pharmacy or grocery store. I also take a small scoop of pink Himalayan salt to cause an uptick in natremia (salt content of blood). The body corrects this hypernatremia by means of osmosis, pulling extracellular water into the vasculature, forcing the veins to expand even further (Orlov & Mongin, 2007). Obviously, none of this will be effective unless you are properly hydrated, so make sure to pound water throughout the day.

Drying Out

Equally important as increasing your intravascular water content is decreasing your interstitial water content, commonly referred to as water weight. Because preventing this water weight is so essential to bringing out the details of your physique, you should be using sodium-free seasoning on everything you eat (aside from the pink Himalayan salt before your workout). You should also be consuming half (if any) the number of egg yolks that you eat when bulking and adding three or four egg whites to supplement the loss of protein. Yolks contain several essential vitamins and minerals, as well as three grams of protein (equivalent to the amount of protein in one egg white), but they contain far too much fat and sodium to be included in a cutting diet. The only issue is that, similar to the NBA, the whites provide considerably less flavor. Thankfully, you're a grown man who has control over his emotions, so sacrificing a bit of taste will be a nonissue.

To aid in preventing this water weight accumulation, as oxymoronic as it sounds, you should be INCREASING your water consumption. As your body dehydrates, a cascade of chemical reactions triggers your adrenal cortex to release aldosterone. This powerful corticosteroid hormone causes your kidneys to reabsorb extra sodium, which water then follows via osmosis (Orlov & Mongin, 2007). After rehydration is achieved, this aldosterone causes the body to store some of its water in the subcutaneous space (between the skin and muscle) to serve as a reservoir in the event of future dehydration spells (Orlov & Mongin, 2007). As impressive as this process may be in the context of evolutionary biology, it undoubtedly serves as a detriment to building an aesthetic physique. If you simply remain at optimum hydration status, your body has no reason to store this extra water.

Filling your stomach with added water will also help ease the hunger pangs you are sure to experience during the low-carb days. Chewing ice cubes or pieces of sugar-free gum are other methods of distracting yourself, as is brushing your teeth. In the meantime, try to enjoy the hunger pangs in the same way that you enjoy a deep triceps burn in the gym. It'll be gone in ten minutes, and your summer shreds will thank you soon enough. And for the love of God, stop eating all that sugar. You're not nine years old anymore, Timmy; having the jawline of a snowman stopped being cute when you could tie your own shoe laces. Act like an adult for once in your miserable life, and maybe we can make some progress out here.

Rage, Rage Against the Dying of the Light

That's all I got, boys. I know it seems like I've been hard on you, but it's only because I truly believe that anyone can improve their physique, and that doing so does not have to consume your life. Most of my friends would describe me as one of the most annoyingly happy people they've ever met, but I can assure you that I have my rough patches just like anyone else. While there certainly are countless avenues to derive confidence, my body has always been among the most effective means for me to pull myself out of a dark headspace. If this book manages to help even a handful of you transform your frame and lift your spirits in the process, then all of my efforts will have been worthwhile. Whether you believe it or not, the body of your dreams is within your grasp. Now that you know what to do, the onus is on you. Apply what I have taught you, push yourself to the absolute limit day in and day out, and I promise that you will be happy with the results. God speed, men. See you next summer.

References

Artioli GG, Gualano B, Smith A, Stout J, Lancha AH Jr. (2010). "Role of beta-alanine supplementation on muscle carnosine and exercise performance." *Medicine & Science in Sports & Exercise* 42(6), 1162-1163.

Brown, Lee & The National Strength and Conditioning Association. (2007). *Strength Training.* Champaign, Il.: Human Kinetics

Burgomaster KA, Hughes SC, Heigenhauser GJ, Bradwell SN & Gibala MJ (2005). "Six sessions of sprint interval training increases muscle oxidative potential and cycle endurance capacity in humans." *Journal of Applied Physiology*, 98, 1985-1990.

Gibala MJ & McGee SL (2008). "Metabolic adaptations to short-term high-intensity interval training: a little pain for a lot of gain?" *Exercise & Sport Sciences Reviews* 36, 58-63.

Golini J (2015). "The effect of an alkaline buffered creatine (Kre-Alkalyn®), on cell membrane behavior, protein synthesis, and cisplatin-mediated cellular toxicity." *Integrative Molecular Medicine*, 2(3): 214-218.

Hall, Matthew DO; Trojian, Thomas H. MD, FACSM (2013). "Creatine Supplementation." *Current Sports Medicine Reports* 12(4): 240-244.

Helms ER, Aragon AA, Fitschen PJ (2014). "Evidence-based recommendations for natural bodybuilding contest preparation: nutrition and supplementation." *Journal of the International Society of Sports Nutrition* 11(20). Online. https://www.ncbi.nlm.nih.gov/pmc/articles/PMC4033492/

Kreider RB, Kalman DS, Antonio J, Zeigenfuss TN, Wildman R, Collins R, Candow DG, Kleiner SM, Almada AL & Lopez HL (2017). "International Society of Sports Nutrition position stand: safety and efficacy of creatine supplementation in exercise, sport, and medicine." *Journal of the International Society of Sports Nutrition* 14(8). Online: https://jissn.biomedcentral.com/articles/10.1186/s12970-017-0173-z

Orlov SN & Mongin AA (2007). "Salt-sensing mechanisms in blood pressure regulation and hypertension." *American Journal of Physiology, Heart and Circulatory Physiology* 293(4): 2039-2053.

Rakobowchuk M, Tanguay S, Burgomaster KA, Howarth KR, Gibala MJ & MacDonald MJ (2008). "Sprint interval and traditional endurance training induce similar improvements in peripheral arterial stiffness and flow-mediated dilation in healthy humans". *American Journal of Physiology, Regulatory Integrative and Comparative Physiology* 295, R236-R242.

Robson, David. 2/19/2019. *Bodybuilding.com*. Online. https://www.bodybuilding.com/fun/dorian_yates_training_insight.htm

Rooney KJ, Herbert RD, & Balnave, RJF. "Fatigue contributes to the strength training stimulus." Medicine & Science in Sports & Exercise 26: 1160-1164, 1994.

CPSIA information can be obtained
at www.ICGtesting.com
Printed in the USA
JSHW011117011119
2191JS00004B/29